漫画中药故事系列
Chinese Medicines
in Cartoon Series

智用中药

（汉英对照）

Tales of Creative Use and TCM
(Chinese-English)

杨柏灿　**主编**
Edited by Yang Baican

杨熠文　晋　永　鲍思思　祝建龙　◎**文/译**
Paperwork by Yang Yiwen, Jin Yong, Bao Sisi, Zhu Jianlong

孔珏莹　夏瑜桢　金潇逸　◎**绘**
Brushwork by Kong Jueying, Xia Yuzhen, Jin Xiaoyi

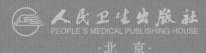
人民卫生出版社
PEOPLE'S MEDICAL PUBLISHING HOUSE
·北 京·

图书在版编目（CIP）数据

智用中药：汉英对照 / 杨柏灿主编 . —北京：人民卫生出版社，2021.3

（漫画中药故事系列）

ISBN 978-7-117-31331-5

Ⅰ.①智… Ⅱ.①杨… Ⅲ.①中药材–普及读物–汉、英 Ⅳ.①R282-49

中国版本图书馆 CIP 数据核字（2021）第 038065 号

| 人卫智网 | www.ipmph.com | 医学教育、学术、考试、健康，购书智慧智能综合服务平台 |
| 人卫官网 | www.pmph.com | 人卫官方资讯发布平台 |

漫画中药故事系列——智用中药（汉英对照）

Manhua Zhongyao Gushi Xilie——Zhiyong Zhongyao（Han-Ying Duizhao）

主　　编：	杨柏灿
出版发行：	人民卫生出版社（中继线 010-59780011）
地　　址：	北京市朝阳区潘家园南里 19 号
邮　　编：	100021
E - mail：	pmph @ pmph.com
购书热线：	010-59787592　010-59787584　010-65264830
印　　刷：	北京顶佳世纪印刷有限公司
经　　销：	新华书店
开　　本：	889×1194　1/24　印张：2.5
字　　数：	73 千字
版　　次：	2021 年 3 月第 1 版
印　　次：	2021 年 4 月第 1 次印刷
标准书号：	ISBN 978-7-117-31331-5
定　　价：	46.00 元

打击盗版举报电话：010-59787491　E-mail：WQ @ pmph.com

质量问题联系电话：010-59787234　E-mail：zhiliang @ pmph.com

序言

Foreword

由上海中医药大学杨柏灿教授主编的《漫画中药故事系列》由人民卫生出版社出版了。这也是杨教授十年来从事中医药文化研究、作品创作和开展中医药文化普及工作的又一力作。

中医药是中国优秀传统文化的代表，凝聚着深邃的中国古代哲学智慧和科学文明的精髓。在抗击新冠肺炎疫情中，中医药发挥了突出的作用，引起世人的高度关注。国家的重视、社会的认同和关注，使中医药的发展迎来了前所未有的大好时机。抓住这一千载难逢的契机，做好中医药的传承与创新、推广与普及工作，是每一位中医药工作者义不容辞的责任。

做好中医药的传承、创新与弘扬，首先重在传承，只有真正做好传承，将中医药的精气神传承下来，才有可能不断创新、发展、弘扬。要做好中医药的传承，除了专业院校的教学以及师承以外，在全社会开展中医药知识的普及推广是一项十分重要的工作，特别是重视"从娃娃抓起"，从小就让我们的孩子沐浴中医药知识的阳光雨露，领略中医药世界的奥秘，感受中国传统文化的伟大，树立文化自信，使之入心入脑，有助于增强孩子们的民族自豪感，激发爱国情怀。

Chinese Medicines in Cartoon Series compiled by Professor Yang Baican from Shanghai University of Traditional Chinese Medicine (SHTCM) is published by People's Medical Publishing House. It is a masterpiece by Professor Yang after his 10-year study on, writing about and popularization of Chinese medicine culture.

Traditional Chinese medicine (TCM) is representative of traditional Chinese culture, where lies the wisdom of ancient Chinese philosophy and the essence of scientific civilization. In the fight against COVID-19 epidemic, TCM has been playing an important role and attracts a lot of attention. Valued by the nation and accepted and followed with interest by the society, TCM has an unprecedented opportunity for development. It is a duty for every TCM worker to seize this opportunity and perform well in inheritance, innovation, promotion and popularization of TCM.

To inherit, innovate and carry forward TCM, inheritance is the first and foremost. TCM can be innovated, developed and carried forward only when it is inherited properly with its essence handed down. For inheritance of TCM, besides teachings in professional schools and from a master to his/her apprentices, it is important to popularize TCM knowledge in the whole society, with focus on "Starts with children". Let our children bathe in the sunshine of TCM knowledge, get to know the mystery of TCM and feel the magnificence of traditional Chinese culture, so that they can have cultural confidence, which helps enhance their sense of national pride and inspire their love for the country.

近年来，一些有识之士已开展了卓有成效的"中医药走进中小学"的工作，受到了广泛的关注和认同。伴随着国家综合实力的增强，我国国际社会地位的提升，中医药的国际影响力也日益扩大。重视中医药走向国际，弘扬中国传统文化，不但有利于提升我国文化软实力，而且也有益于中医药为全人类造福。

杨柏灿教授是上海中医药大学从事中药学教学的教师。他在完成中医药的医、教、研工作之余，十年来致力于中医药知识的推广与普及工作，在国内最早开设了中药慕课课程《走近中药》《杏林探宝——带你走进中药》《杏林探宝——认知中药》《中药学》《中药知多少》以及微视频《中药知识——走进中小学》。其中《杏林探宝——认知中药》上线美国 Coursera 平台，受众人群遍及 80 余个国家和地区，学习人数达 10 余万人次。同时，杨教授笔耕不辍，六年来先后出版了中医药通识读本《药缘文化——中药与文化的交融》《药名文化——中药与文化的交融》，连续三年出版了《本草光阴——中药养生文化日历》，在社会上产生一定的影响。

In recent years, men of sight have carried out projects of "Introducing TCM into middle and primary schools", which is widely concerned and approved. With enhancement of the overall national strength and the elevated status of China in the international community, TCM has an increasingly large international influence. Paying attention to international communication of TCM and carrying forward traditional Chinese culture can not only strengthen the cultural soft power of China, but also bring benefit for all mankind.

The author is a professor in Chinese medicines in SHTCM. After finishing his work as a doctor, teacher and researcher in TCM, he has been dedicated to promotion and popularization of TCM knowledge for nearly a decade. He is the first to provide MOOCs on Chinese medicines in China, including *Get Closer to Chinese Medicines*, *Hunt for Treasure in Apricot Grove — Bring You Closer to Chinese Medicines*, *Hunt for Treasure in Apricot Grove — Get to Know Chinese Medicines*, *Traditional Chinese Pharmacology* and *What Do You Know About Chinese Medicines*, as well as a micro video of *Knowledge about Chinese Medicines — Introduced into Middle and Primary Schools*. Among them, *Hunt for Treasure in Apricot Grove — Get to Know Chinese Medicines* is available online on Coursera, with audience from more than 80 countries and regions and learned by over 100,000 person-time. At the same time, Professor Yang has been writing continuously. In recent six years, he has published books on TCM including *Medicine Culture—Blending of Chinese Medicines and Culture* and *Medicine Name Culture—Blending of Chinese Medicines and Culture* and has published *Time and Chinese Materia Medica—Health Culture Calendar with Chinese Medicines*, which has a certain social impact.

《漫画中药故事系列》突破了目前市面上单纯以文字讲中药故事，或是将中药故事与中药知识相割离的作品形式，遍查古籍，选取有史实依据、民众知晓度高、具有深厚中国传统文化底蕴的中药故事，通过生动形象的漫画和精练朴实的语言，讲解中药故事，向世人展示中药知识与中国多元优秀传统文化的交融。读者在赏读本丛书时，不但能了解常用的中药知识，还能在不知不觉中接受中国传统文化的熏陶。本丛书的文字部分采用中英文对照的形式，益于中医药在国际上传播，同时也使中小学生在阅读漫画、接受中医药知识之余，提升英语的阅读能力。

本丛书的出版发行对于中医药的推广、普及势必有一定的促进作用，期待杨柏灿教授团队能不断有新的作品问世。

上海市卫生健康委员会副主任
上海市中医药管理局副局长
上海中医药学会会长
原上海中医药大学副校长

胡鸿毅

2020 年 9 月

Chinese Medicines in Cartoon Series gets rid of the layout of telling stories about Chinese medicines in words alone or separating the stories from the knowledge. The author has consulted ancient books and selected the stories that are based on historical facts, well known among people and deeply rooted in traditional Chinese culture. The stories about Chinese medicines are told through vivid cartoons and in simple language. They show the world the blending of knowledge about Chinese medicines with traditional Chinese culture, so that the reader can not only know about Chinese medicines, but also feel the charm of traditional Chinese culture. The text part of the series of books is in both Chinese and English to promote international spread of TCM, and additionally, the students in middle and primary schools can have their English reading ability improved while reading the cartoons and learning about Chinese medicines.

Publishing and distribution of this series of books will surely give an impetus to the promotion and popularization of TCM and I look forward to more works by the team led by Professor Yang Baican.

Deputy director, Shanghai Municipal Health Commission

Deputy director, Shanghai Municipal Administrator of Traditional Chinese Medicine

President, Shanghai Association of Traditional Chinese Medicine

Former vice-president, Shanghai University of Traditional Chinese Medicine

Hu Hongyi

Sep, 2020

醫者善聽本寧言
中藥智慧綿千年
采藥順天育應地
同源異位亦當親
佩書釀技任藥引
用藥育術功效顯

前言

Preface

随着我国综合实力的不断提高和国际地位的日益提升，文化软实力建设、树立文化自信，已成为国家的发展战略。习近平总书记指出"中医药学凝聚着深邃的哲学智慧和中华民族几千年的健康养生理念及其实践经验，是中国古代科学的瑰宝，也是打开中华文明宝库的钥匙"，高屋建瓴地概括了中医药在传统文化中具有不可替代的地位及其所具有的鲜明的文化特征。

《漫画中药故事系列》以历史悠久、扎根于中华大地、深植于大众心灵的中药为切入点，通过具有史料记载、民间知晓度高的典故传说，采用形象生动的漫画形式，传播中药知识，弘扬传统文化。丛书共分四册，既可独立成书又前后互为关联。

第一册《名医药传》：从中药雅称、药物应用、功效发现，介绍家喻户晓的名医名家治疗顽苛痼疾、疑难杂症的故事。

第二册《君药传奇》：从药名来历、药物应用等方面，介绍中药与古代君王间的趣闻典故以及民间医药高手不畏权贵、巧用中药的故事。

With its increasing comprehensive strength and growing status in the world, China's cultural soft power along with cultural confidence turns to renascent tendency. Chinese President Xi Jinping, once claimed that "Traditional Chinese medical theory is the gem of ancient Chinese science and philosophy, and also a key to the treasure of Chinese civilization", reconfirming the irreplaceable position and distinct feature of traditional Chinese medicine (TCM) in our culture.

Chinese Medicines in Cartoon Series aims at spreading knowledge of TCM and promoting our national culture. The series takes the well-known herbs as entry, tells fact-based tales and illustrates stories with pictures in comic format. The series includes four books, each being a sub-topic of TCM.

Book I *Tales of Doctors and TCM*: stories about miscellaneous and critical cases, mainly from the aspects of herbs' poetic names and efficacy.

Book II *Tales of Emperors and TCM*: stories about emperors and herbs, mainly from the aspects of herbs' naming and efficacy.

第三册《品读中药》：从汤羹、酒与豆腐发明的故事，介绍中药与饮食文化的渊源，体现药食同源的特性；通过益母草、王不留行、远志等中药名称来历的典故，体现中药药名的文化内涵。

第四册《智用中药》：从药物生长环境、采摘时节、药用部位、应用方式等对药效的影响，体现古今医药学家认识自然、应用自然的智慧。

随着国家对中医药工作日益重视以及在这次抗击新冠肺炎疫情中，中医药不可或缺的作用，重视做好中医药的传承、创新及推广已成为全社会的共识。特别是近年来，越来越多人意识到，要做好中医药的传承应该从小抓起，要重视中医药走进中小学的工作。正是在这样的大背景下，本团队经过 3 年多的努力，在人民卫生出版社的大力支持下，完成了以传播中药知识、弘扬传统文化为宗旨的漫画中药故事系列丛书。期望本丛书的出版发行，能有益于中医药知识和传统文化的传播。

Book Ⅲ *Tales of Food and TCM*: stories about herbs and diet through the invention of soup, wine and tofu; stories about herbs and its name origin through the naming of motherwort, polygala, etc.

Book Ⅳ *Tales of Creative Use and TCM*: stories about herbs and efficacy, mainly from the aspects of herbs' living environment, growing seasons, plant parts and application.

With the increasing emphasis on the traditional Chinese medical theory and its indispensable role in the combat against COVID-19, the whole society has reached the consensus that the traditional Chinese medical theory should be inherited, innovated as well as promoted. In recent years, more and more people have realized that the inheritance of TCM should be cultivated since childhood and that TCM should be introduced into elementary education stage. Thanks to People's Medical Publishing House, our team, after more than three years' constant efforts, has completed this series of comic books on TCM. We are hoping that Chinese medicine and traditional Chinese culture can be promoted after its publication.

考虑到中西方文化背景的不同，在英语翻译上侧重于意译，而非直译，部分内容及标题中英文有所不同，须结合具体故事情节予以理解。

本丛书适用于广大中医药爱好者，特别是中小学生。同时，本丛书中英对照的形式也有助于在国际上传播、宣传中医药知识和中国传统文化，推动中医药国际化。

Owning to the cultural differences between the East and the West, some parts of the stories have been translated sense-for-sense instead word-for-word.

This series of books is written for Chinese medicine enthusiasts, especially primary and middle school students. Meanwhile, in the form of both Chinese and English, it helps to spread Chinese medicine knowledge and culture so as to promote its internationalization.

《漫画中药故事系列》丛书编委会

Editorial Committee

2020 年 7 月 25 日

July 25, 2020

目录
CATALOG

第一部分
识药之语

中药虽然不会说话，但古人通过药物生长的季节、环境与自身
秉性读懂了药物的语言，发现了药物的功效。

Part I
Listening to the Language of
Medicine

Although traditional Chinese medicine is mute,
the ancients found out the efficacy of the herbs by
understanding the language of them through observing
their growing seasons, studying living environment and
analyzing their own biological characteristics.

甲骨文名缘中药

The Language in Oracle Bone Inscriptions

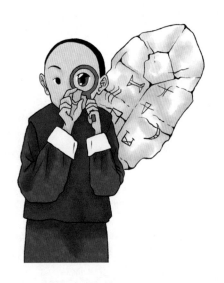

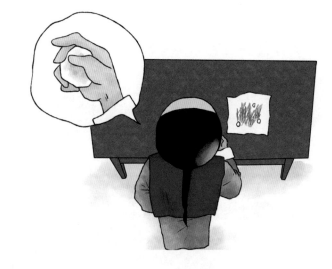

王懿荣是清代著名的金石学家，首先发现了甲骨文字。而这段发现经历却是得益于两味中药。

Wang Yirong was a famous scholar on epigraphy in the Qing Dynasty who first discovered the inscriptions on bones and tortoise shells. However, his great discovery had some relation with two traditional Chinese medicines.

清光绪年间，时任国子监祭酒的王懿荣患了疟疾。

During the reign of Emperor Guangxu of the Qing Dynasty, Wang Yirong, a libationer in the imperial college, caught malaria.

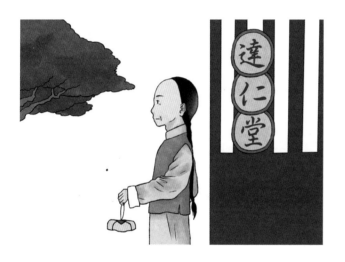

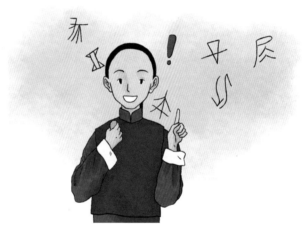

在经大夫诊疗之后，他从达仁堂中药店买回了一剂治病的中药。

Having been diagnosed, Wang bought a dose of prescription from Daren Tang, a Chinese pharmacy.

在煎药过程中，王懿荣无意中发现了一味叫"龙骨"的中药上隐隐约约刻了一些符号。

While decocting the medicine, Wang Yirong accidentally found some signs vaguely engraved on a kind of medicine called "Longgu (animal fossil fragments)".

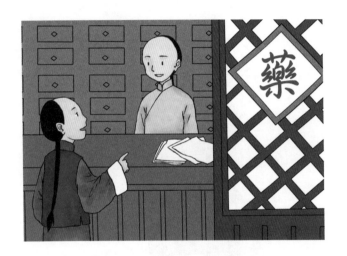

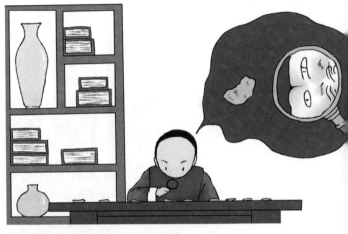

身为金石学家的他，敏锐地意识到这龙骨上所刻的可能是一些古代的符号。

于是他派人到药店，以每片 2 两银子的高价，把药店里刻有符号的龙骨全买了下来。

Being an epigraphist, instinctively he sensed that these signs might be some ancient symbols conveying special meanings.

So he had all the Longgu with symbols collected at a high price of 2 liang (an ancient Chinese monetary unit) each piece.

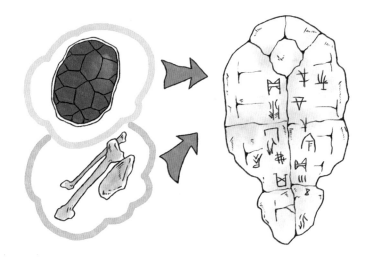

他开始对这些符号进行仔细的研究，终于从《周礼》和《史记》中找到了线索。这些文字正是秦汉之前的上古文字。

Then he began to study these symbols carefully, and finally he got some clues from *Rites of Zhou* and *Historical Records*. These symbols were actually the ancient characters before Qin and Han Dynasties.

自此以后，不仅是龙骨，又有许多文字在另一味中药——龟甲上得以发现，因而这些中国最古老的文字被称之为"甲骨文"，而王懿荣也因此被认作为"甲骨文"之父。

Since then, not only on the Longgu, but also on the Guijia (tortoise shells)—another kind of traditional Chinese medicine, have many characters been found. Therefore, these China's oldest characters are called "oracle bone inscriptions", and accordingly, Wang Yirong is regarded as "the father" of it.

龟甲、龙骨功效
The Efficacy of Tortoise Shell, and Fossil Fragments

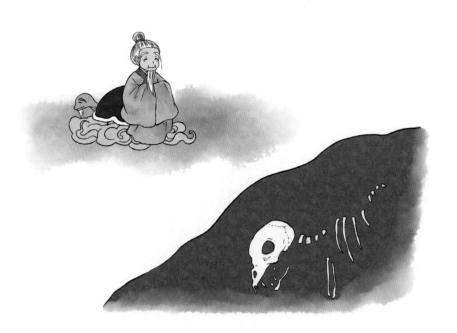

功效分析

文中的龙骨是古代大型哺乳动物骨骼的化石。其往往深埋于地底深处，而有着能够长期保存、不易腐败的特点，因此被古人选作篆刻文字的媒介。也是因其长埋地底，历经千年，古人认为其吸收自然界的精华，故而不同于普通骨骼，具有重镇的特性，既能重镇镇静安神，又可重镇平肝潜阳。龟甲是龟的腹甲与背甲，坚硬而牢固，保护其免受外界因素的侵袭，古人将其用于刻写文字也是源于此。同时，中医认为寿命与肾的关系密切，而龟又是长寿的象征，故龟甲长于补肾，具有益肾健骨的功效。

Efficacy Analysis

Longgu in the above story are the fossil of ancient large mammal bones, often buried deeply underground, so they can be preserved for a long time without decay. Therefore, they were chosen as the medium of seal cutting by ancient people. The ancients believed that Longgu, absorbing the essence of nature, were different from ordinary bones. Having characteristics of tranquilization with heavy nature, they could not only calm down the nerves, but also the liver, and suppress yang. Guijia is the tortoise's ventral and dorsal carapace, which is hard and solid to protect it from external dangers. It was used for writing characters by the ancients as well. According to traditional Chinese medical theory, life expectancy is believed to be closely related to kidney, and tortoise is a symbol of longevity, so Guijia is good at nourishing kidney, strengthening sinews and bones.

顺天应时采中药
The Language in Seasons

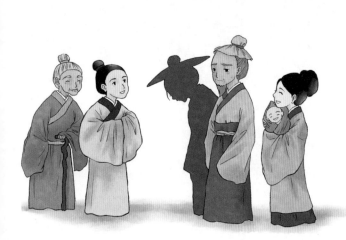
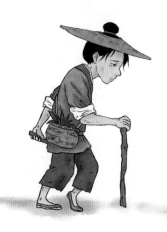
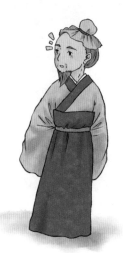

华佗是东汉末年著名的医学家，医术精湛，总能妙手回春，被后人誉为"神医"，但是有一天，他却遇到了一个难题。

Hua Tuo was a famous medical expert in the late Eastern Han Dynasty. He had excellent medical skills and was always able to bring his patients back to life, so he was praised as a "miracle working doctor" by later generations. But one day, he had a problem.

三月的一日，一位以挖野菜为生的穷苦樵夫拄着拐杖来找华佗："先生，请您给我治治吧。"华佗见其面容憔悴，身目俱黄，便知其人得了黄疸病。

One day in March, a poor woodcutter, who made a living by digging wild vegetables, went on crutch to Hua Tuo, "Sir, please save me." On seeing his gaunt face and yellow eyes, Hua Tuo knew at once that he had got jaundice.

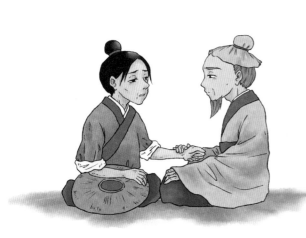

华佗上前为其诊脉，诊后却皱着眉头，无奈地摇了摇头说："这个病，我也无能为力啊。"

Hua Tuo came forward to examine his pulse. After the examination, he frowned, shook his head helplessly and said, "I'm so sorry. I can do nothing to help you."

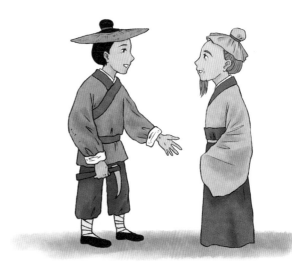

半年后秋日里的一天，华佗又巧遇这位樵夫，见其面色红润，精神抖擞，华佗诧异不已，急忙问道："你的病是哪位先生治好的？"

Half a year later on an autumn day, Hua Tuo happened to meet the woodcutter again. Seeing his rosy complexion and vigorous spirit, Hua Tuo was surprised, "Who has cured your disease?" he asked eagerly.

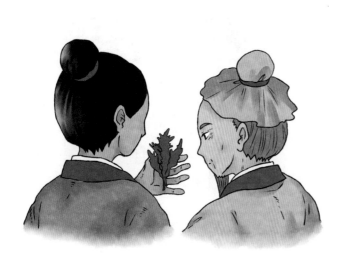

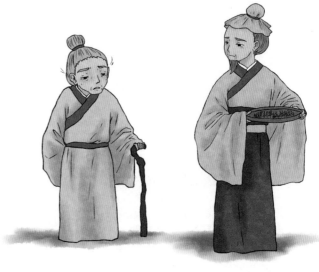

樵夫说："我没有再找先生看病，只是在春天的这几个月吃了这种野菜。"说完便拿出了野菜给华佗看，华佗一看便知这是茵陈，心想或许茵陈是治疗黄疸的特效药。

"Not a single doctor have I visited!" answered the woodcutter. "In fact, I ate this wild vegetable in the spring months. " He took out some wild herbs and showed them to Hua Tuo. Hua Tuo knew at a glance that this was Yinchen (*Artemisia scoparia*). He thought perhaps these might be the specific medicine working for jaundice.

于是，华佗便采了一些茵陈回去，用来治疗其他黄疸的病人，可是都没有获得疗效。

Therefore, Hua Tuo took some Yinchen back. He also tried the herb to treat patients with jaundice, but got no effect.

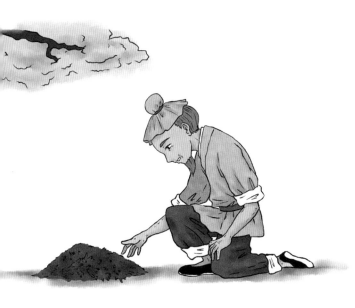

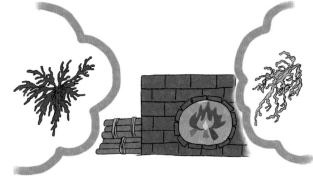

华佗不解，仔细思索后突然醒悟到，这可能这和季节有关。

Hua Tuo was puzzled. After careful thinking, he suddenly came to realise that this might be related to the season.

于是等到第二年开春三月，华佗又去采了一些茵陈，给黄疸的病人服用，果然药到病除。因而，在民间有这样一句歌诀，趣味地描写道："三月茵陈四月蒿，五月过了当柴烧。"

Then in the following spring, Hua Tuo went in March to collect some Yinchen and prescribed them to patients with jaundice. As was expected, this time the medicine worked. In fact, there is a folk song saying: "Yinchen, a good medicine in March, a kind of vegetable in April, but just firewood after May."

茵陈功效
The Efficacy of *Artemisia scoparia*

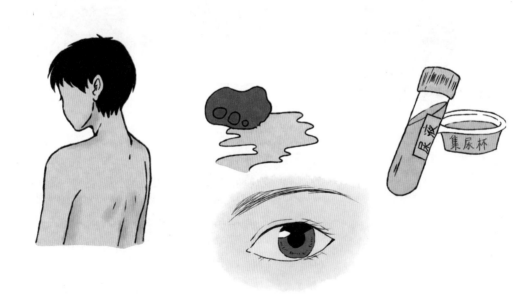

功效分析

黄疸是以身黄，目黄，小便黄为症状特点的疾病。中医认为黄疸为湿热蕴结，胆汁外溢所致，故治疗既要利湿给邪有去路，又要利胆使胆汁循于常道。茵陈既能利胆退黄，又可利湿退黄，自古便是治疗黄疸的要药和专药。但就如文中古老歌诀中所描写的那样，"三月茵陈四月蒿，五月过了当柴烧"，时间赋予了药材千变万化的特性，即使是治疗黄疸的专药茵陈，采摘时间不同，其疗效也有云泥之别。故历代医家对药物的采摘时间有明确的要求，如桑叶以霜打后为佳，橘皮以陈久者为良。这便是中药文化中的时间智慧。

Efficacy Analysis

Jaundice is a disease characterized by yellow body surface, yellow eyes and yellow urine. Traditional Chinese medical theory believes that jaundice is caused by damp-heat accumulation and bile overflow. Therefore, the treatment should not only promote dampness to give pathogenic factors a way, but also promote bile to follow the normal path. Yinchen can not only normalize the gallbladder's disorder, but also eliminate dampness to relieve jaundice. Yinchen has been an important and special medicine for the treatment of jaundice since ancient times. However, as described in the ancient verse, time endows medicinal materials with ever-changing characteristics. Special medicine for jaundice as Yinchen is, its curative effect can be totally different if collected in different months. Therefore, physicians of all dynasties have clear requirements for medicine picking. For example, mulberry leaves are better after frost beating and tangerine peel nicer after being stored for a long time. This shows the wisdom of time in Chinese medical culture.

生长环境育中药

The Language in Growing Environment

李時珍

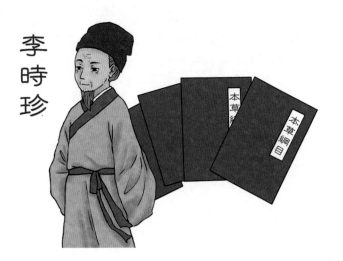

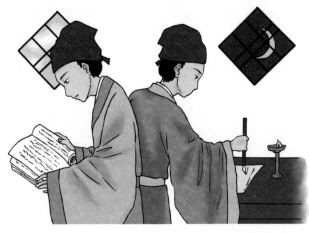

明代李时珍历时二十七年在其晚年完成了药物学巨著《本草纲目》。然而这位医学大家却曾在年轻时经历了生死考验。

In the Ming Dynasty, Li Shizhen worked 27 years on his magnum opus *Compendium of Materia Medica* before final completion in his later years. However, this medical expert once experienced the test of life and death when he was young.

据李时珍回忆，当时弱冠之年的他正为金榜题名而废寝忘食，日夜苦读。

According to Li Shizhen's memory, he was then working hard day and night preparing for the national examination.

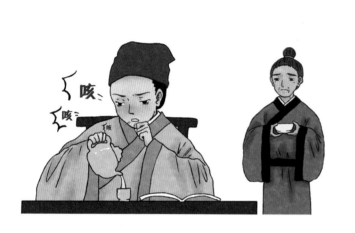

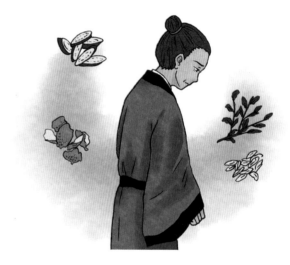

不过由于思劳过度，李时珍患上感冒，咳嗽不止，皮肤犹如火燎。

Unfortunately, due to overstrain, Li Shizhen suffered from a cold. He coughed constantly and his skin was like burning.

李时珍的父亲李言闻也是当时的一位名医，他断其为肺热所困，便让儿子服下了芦根、甘草、知母等许多清肺热之药，却都不见效。

Li Shizhen's father, Li Yanwen, was also a famous doctor at that time. He diagnosed his son as being trapped by lung heat, so he let him take many lung-heat-clearing drugs such as reed rhizome, licorice root and anemarrhena rhizome, but none worked.

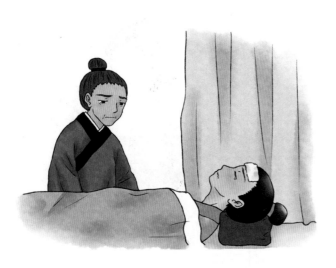

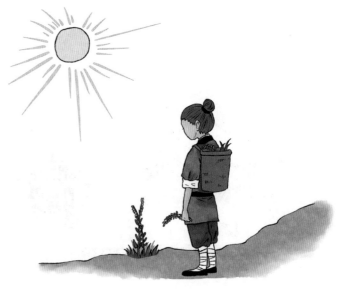

眼见儿子病情一天天加重，寝食俱废，做父亲的可谓是心急如焚。

偶然一次采药过程中，父亲发现在向阳山坡阳光的炙烤下，有一株植物却生长茂盛，走近一看，发现这便是黄芩，于是马上联想到黄芩长于清热的特性。

Seeing his son get weaker day by day, the father was extremely demented.

One day on his usual herb-collecting journey, the father found a flourishing plant on a sunny hillside under the hot burning sunlight. When seeing closer, he recognized that it was Huangqin (*Scutellaria baicalensis*). Immediately he thought of its feature of clearing heat.

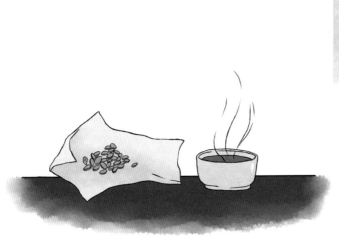

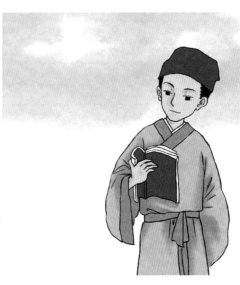

回到家，父亲便立马取了黄芩片一两煎汤，给李时珍服下。

第二日，李时珍果然热退，咳嗽也好了大半，继而又投入科举备考之中。

On arriving home, he took one liang of Huangqin for decoction and gave it to the son.

On the following day, Li Shizhen felt much better: his fever was gone as expected and the cough was much relieved as well. So after recovery, Li Shizhen went on with his exam preparation.

黄芩功效
The Efficacy of *Scutellaria baicalensis*

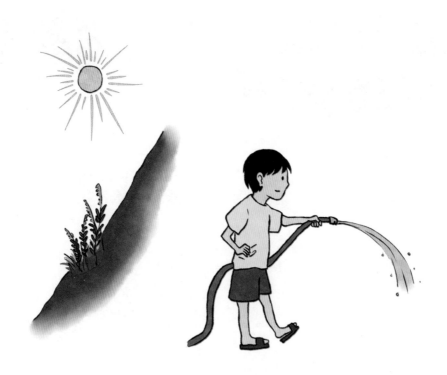

功效分析

黄芩多生长于干旱的向阳山坡的草丛中。不难想象，向阳山坡在太阳的炙烤下，连石头都会烫手，植物怎么可能生长呢？因而，能在这种环境下生长的植物必然具有抗热、耐旱的特性。抗热而性寒可清热，耐旱而味苦可燥湿，故黄芩的主要功效为清热泻火，燥湿解毒。故事中李时珍高热不退、肌肤如灼，是一派热毒壅肺的表现，父亲用了甘草、芦根等清热的药物，虽大方向并不错，但清热的力量不够。黄芩苦寒之性重，清泄之力强，尤善清泄肺热，故以此治疗自然药到病除。

Efficacy Analysis

Huangqin mostly grows in the grass on the dry sunny hillside. It is not hard to imagine that even stones on sunny hillsides are burning, but how can plants grow? Those plants growing there must be heat-resistant and drought enduring. "Heat-resistant" implies its cold nature that can clear heat; "drought enduring" implies its bitter taste that can dry dampness, so the main effects of Huangqin are clearing heat and purging fire, drying dampness and detoxifying. In the story, Li Shizhen's persistent high fever, burning skin were manifestations of heat toxin accumulated in lung. His father used drugs such as licorice and reed rhizome to clear heat. Although those were the right medicine, they were not strong enough. Huangqin is bitter and cold in nature and strong in clearing and discharging lung heat. Naturally it was able to cure in the story.

同源异位辨中药
The Language in Plant Parts

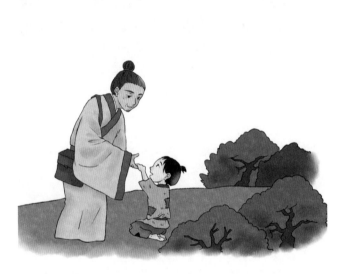

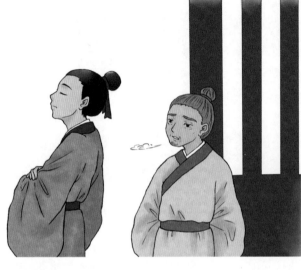

有一天，一个老郎中出门采药，发现一个小孩在路边甚是可怜，便收养在身边，认他做徒弟，教他医术。

One day, a senior doctor was going out for medicine collecting when he accidentally found a poor child on the roadside. Full of mercy, he took the child as an apprentice and taught him medical skills.

谁想，这个徒弟长大后很是狂妄，才学会一点皮毛，就看不起师傅了。

When the apprentice grew up, he became very arrogant, and even began to look down upon his master though he had hardly learned anything.

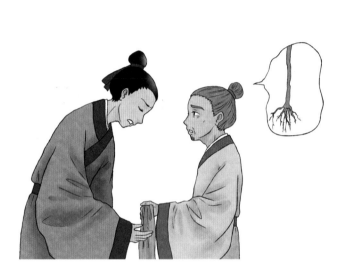

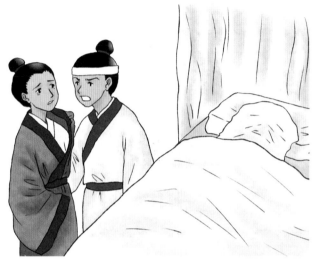

师傅伤透了心，同意其另立门户，临走前提醒他麻黄这味药千万不能用错，它的茎是发汗的，它的根是止汗的。但是徒弟丝毫不放心上。

Though heartbroken, the master agreed to let him go. Before leaving, the master reminded him that Mahuang (*Ephedra sinica*) must not be used by mistake, for its stem was for sweating while its root for hidroschesis. But the apprentice did not take it to heart.

自此以后，徒弟便开始独自行医。可是好景不长，徒弟因为错用麻黄治死了人。

Since then, the apprentice started practicing medicine by himself. However, it was not long before he killed a patient because of the wrong use of Mahuang.

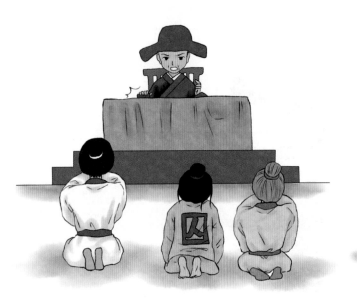

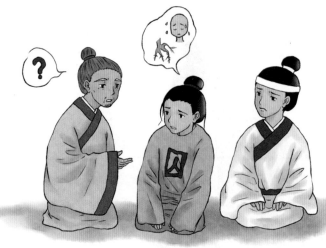

死者家属伤心欲绝，将其告上公堂。县令认为医术不精是师傅教导无方之过，便要求将其师傅抓来，要一并致罪。

The bereaved family was so inconsolable that they sued the apprentice in court. The county magistrate believed that it was the master's responsibility for the apprentice's poor medical skill, so he demanded that his master be arrested and punished together.

师傅再次询问徒弟这药的功效以及病人所患何病。徒弟怯怯地答道："发汗用茎，止汗用根，病人为出汗之病，但我却错用了茎。"

Again the master asked the apprentice about the efficacy of the Mahuang and the very disease the victim had suffered from. The apprentice replied cowardly, "Stem is for sweating, and root is for hidroschesis. The patient suffered from sweating, but I used stems by mistake."

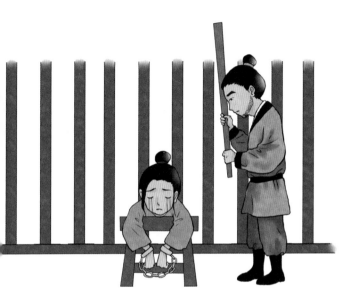

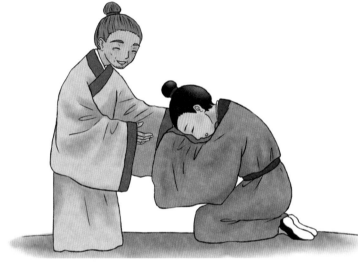

县令听后大怒，命人杖责徒弟四十大板，并判其入狱三年。师傅则被当堂释放。

After hearing this, the county magistrate got furious and ordered the apprentice to be flogged 40 strokes and be sentenced to three years' imprisonment, while the master was released right now.

三年后，徒弟找到师傅，并向师傅认了错，表示要痛改前非，潜心钻研医术。师傅见他诚心悔过，这才把他留下，继续向他传授医道。

Three years later, the apprentice went back to the master and made a sincere apology, saying that he would turn a new leaf and work hard to amend. Seeing his repentance, the master forgave him and continued to teach him.

麻黄功效
The Efficacy of *Ephedra sinica*

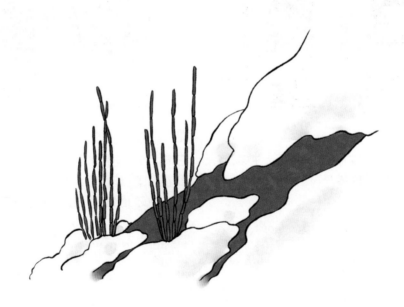

功效分析

麻黄生长于寒冷的西北地区，寒冷的季节常常是冰天雪地。但麻黄具有一个特点，其生长的周围却常年不积雪，故《本草纲目》将其特性归纳为"泄阳"二字，表明麻黄性温热，并且能够将体内的热量向外发散，使得周围冰雪无法堆积。麻黄发汗之力很强，被誉为"发汗解表第一药"，这便是故事中师傅反复叮嘱徒儿务必谨慎使用的原因所在。但一味的发散，势必会损耗自身。因此，麻黄的节和根与麻黄茎功效截然相反，不但不发汗，反而能够收敛止汗，防止其过度辛散，维持着自身的动态平衡。

Efficacy Analysis

Mahuang grows in the cold northwest region, the weather of which is often snowy in cold seasons. However, Mahuang has a characteristic that the soil around it is not covered with snow all the year round. Therefore, the *Compendium of Materia Medica* classifies its characteristic as "draining yang", which indicates that Mahuang is warm in nature and can radiate heat in the body outward, making it impossible for snow or ice to accumulate around it. Therefore, Mahuang is powerful on sweating and is credited with "the strongest medicine for sweating and relieving exterior syndrome". This is why in the story the master repeatedly told his apprentice to use it with great care. Blind sweating will certainly harm the body. The node and root of Mahuang and its stem have completely opposite effects. Instead of sweating, the node and root can restrain sweating, prevent excessive pungent dispersion, and maintain the self-dynamic balance.

第二部分
用药之术

中药并非只有汤剂，也并非所有中药都是天然药物，中药的使用方式中同样蕴藏着许多学问。

Part II
The Skills of Using Medicine

Traditional Chinese medicine comes in the form of more than decoction and natural herbs. There is a lot of profound knowledge in the skillful use of traditional Chinese medicine.

辟秽香囊悬艾草
Fragrant Herbs Preventing Disease

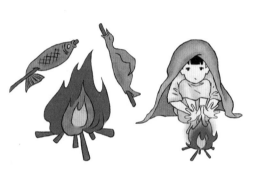
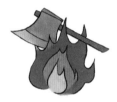
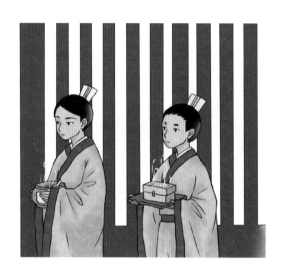

火的应用，在人类文明发展史上具有极其重要的意义，古代民众用火来烹饪美食，依靠火来取暖、冶炼等等。

Fire is of great significance in the development of human civilization. With fire, our ancestors were able to cook, warm, smelt and so on.

古时候，保管和传递火种非常重要，一旦火种遗失，人们便恐面临饥寒交迫的处境。因此，火种往往由专人负责管理。

In ancient times, it was very important to keep and transmit fire. Once the fire died down, people would have to be faced with hunger and cold. Therefore, the fire was often guarded by specific personnel.

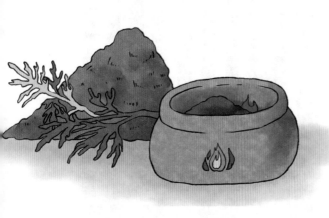

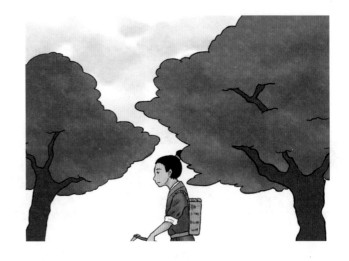

相传当时火种的保存与传递用的是一种中药——
艾叶。

The legend goes that Ai leaves (*Artemisia argyi*),
a traditional Chinese medicine, was used for the
preservation and transmission the fire.

每年端午前后，正是艾生长最旺盛的时期，保管
火种的人会经常上山采集艾叶制成艾绒，以备取
火或保存延续火种之用。

Every year around the Dragon Boat Festival is the
period when Ai grows most vigorously. People in
charge often collected Ai leaves on the mountain to
make moxa, so as to prepare for the fire or preserve it.

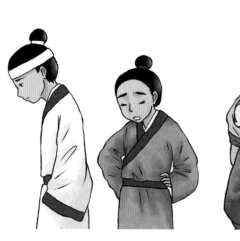
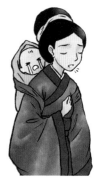
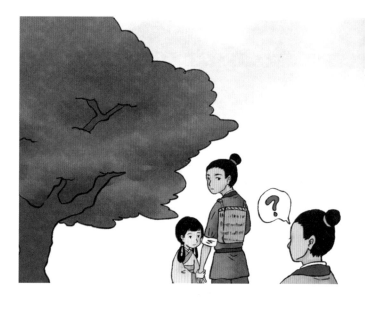

在这段时间，气温逐渐升高，雨水增多，蚊虫滋生，村子部落也往往面临着疾病和瘟疫的侵袭。一旦瘟疫来袭，村子部落里的大部分人都会感染瘟疫而死亡。

During this period, as the temperature gradually increased with more abundant rain, mosquitoes bred in large number. So the villagers were often exposed to diseases and plagues. Once plagues broke out, the majority of the people would be infected and die.

奇怪的是，人们发现每次瘟疫流行时，负责掌管火种的这家人总是安然无恙。

However, the family guarding the fire were always safe and sound every time the plague spread. That greatly surprised the villagers.

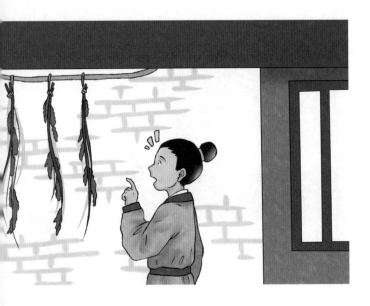

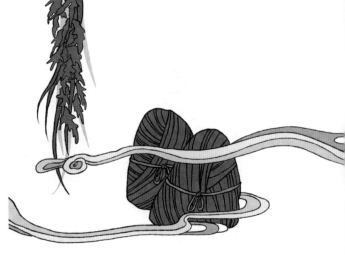

他们仔细检查了这家人与其他人家的不同之处，发现这家人土屋的墙上挂满了艾叶。

They carefully examined the family, focusing on the differences between the family and other households. At last, they found that on the walls of the family's mud hut hung plenty of Ai leaves.

经过人们的反复实践，发现悬挂艾叶确有避免邪气侵害的功效，后来便渐渐演变成端午节悬挂艾叶、佩戴香囊的习俗。

After repeated practice, people came to realize that hanging Ai leaves did have the effect of preventing pathogen from invading. Later, it gradually became a custom of hanging Ai leaves and wearing a fragrant bag during the Dragon Boat Festival.

艾叶功效
The Efficacy of *Artemisia argyi*

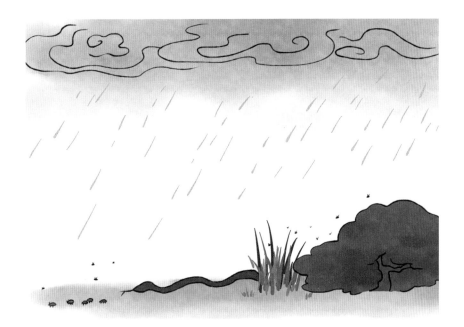

功效分析

端午前后，尤其是江南地区正值梅雨时节，气温升高，雨水增多，环境潮湿，蚊虫滋生，是一些传染病、皮肤病高发的时期。中医认为这与自然界的湿浊秽气相关，而芳香之品可化湿辟秽，艾叶的应用便应运而生。艾叶气味芳香，民间常用艾叶烟熏的方法杀虫驱蚊以防蚊虫叮咬；或将艾叶悬挂在门窗前，并佩戴艾叶制成的香袋以芳香辟秽。另外，艾叶性质温热，除辟秽祛邪外，也可温经散寒，治疗一些寒性痛证。

Efficacy Analysis

Around the Dragon Boat Festival, especially in the south of the Yangtze River, during the plum rains season, the temperature rises, the rain increases, humidity accumulates and mosquitoes breed. As a result, it becomes a period of high incidence of some infectious diseases and skin-related diseases. Traditional Chinese medical theory believes that all those diseases are related to the damp and dirty air in nature, and that fragrant products can resolve dampness and filth. As Aiye has a fragrant smell, people keep off mosquitoes either by using its smoke emitted when burning, or the leaves in front of doors and windows, or wearing fragrant bags with Aiye inside. Aiye is warm in nature. It can dispel filth and pathogenic factors. Besides, it can also warm meridians and dispel cold, so it is often used to treat some cold pain syndromes.

药食相用酿豆豉
Artificial Synthetic Drugs

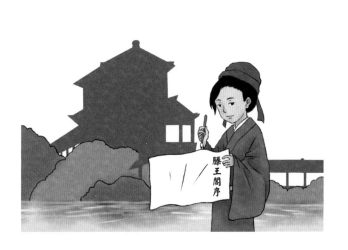

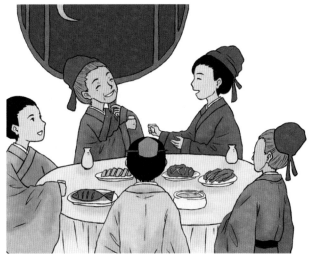

唐代诗人王勃被誉为"初唐四杰"之首，其所著的《滕王阁序》文采斐然，被世人所称道。不过大家是否知道，他与中药还有一段小插曲呢。

Tang Dynasty poet Wang Bo was praised as the No. 1 of the "four outstanding figures in the early Tang Dynasty". His *Preface to the Tengwang Pavilion* was so well-written that it has been praised by generations after generations. However, have you heard of his story with Chinese medicine?

唐上元二年，南昌都督阎伯屿重修滕王阁完成而大宴宾客，为其作序的王勃自然也位列其中。

In the second year of Shangyuan Period in the Tang Dynasty, Yan Boyu, Nanchang Governor, had Tengwang Pavilion rebuilt. After that, he invited guests to a grand banquet. Wang Bo, the writer of the preface for the pavilion, was naturally among them.

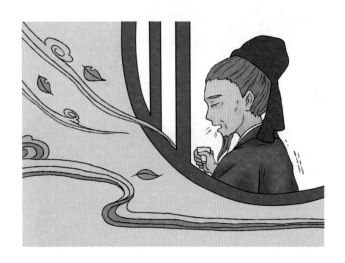

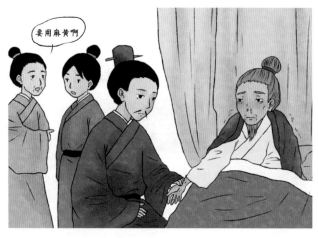

然而连日宴请，阎都督由于贪杯而复感外邪病倒了，只觉浑身怕冷酸疼，汗不得出，于是便请来了当地多位名医诊治。

After several days of banquets, Governor Yan suddenly felt ill due to excessive drinking and external pathogens. He felt cold, sore, and didn't sweat, so he consulted many local doctors.

众医家都认为这是外感风寒所致，其症状与麻黄汤证相似，当以麻黄为君药，发汗解表来治疗。

The doctors said that it was caused by exogenous wind-cold. Since its symptoms were similar to those of Mahuang (*Ephedra sinica*) decoction syndrome, they believed that Mahuang should be used as the monarch drug to treat the disease through sweating and relieving exterior syndrome.

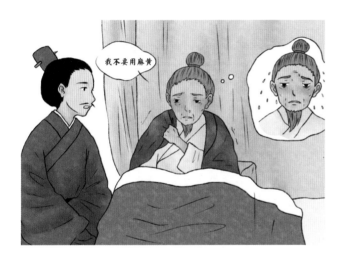

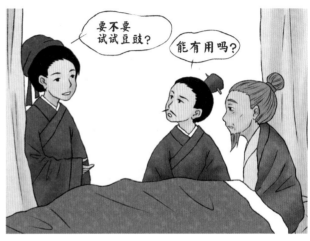

但阎都督也略懂医术，认为麻黄发汗太过，他已年过半百，身体日渐虚弱，恐釜底抽薪，不能承受。

However, Governor Yan, with some knowledge about medical skills, didn't agree with them. He thought that Mahuang was too strong in sweating and his weak body——for he was already above 50 years old——was unable to stand.

这时，王勃见众医家束手无策，就提出用豆豉来治疗。可是大家都不以为然，这小小的豆豉能有多大作用？

Seeing the doctors' wit's end, Wang Bo proposed to treat with Douchi (fermented soya beans). Everybody doubted, "Could these small beans work?"

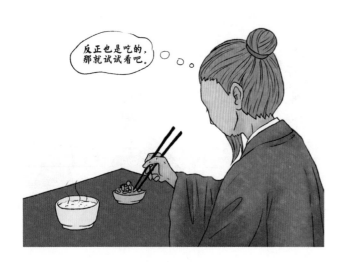

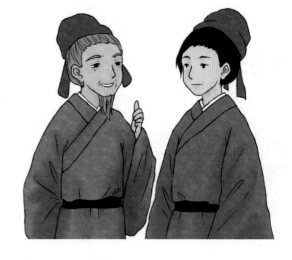

阎都督想，这豆豉也是食物，对身体无碍，王勃又是府上贵宾，不妨试试看吧。

"Douchi is indeed a kind of food, which should not do harm to health," Governor Yan said to himself. "Besides, Wang Bo is a distinguished guest, so I'd better give it a try."

果不其然，阎都督连服三天便微微出了一身汗，过不多久热便退了，不禁又对王勃大加赞赏。

After taking Douchi for three days, Governor Yan was slightly sweaty, and soon the fever was gone. He couldn't help praising Wang Bo again.

豆豉功效
The Efficacy of Fermented Soya Beans

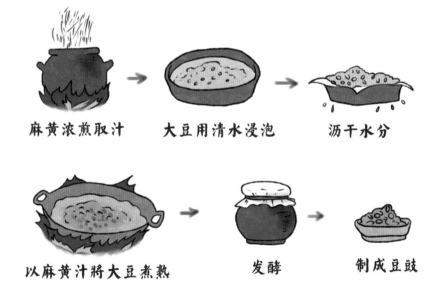

麻黄浓煎取汁   大豆用清水浸泡   沥干水分

以麻黄汁将大豆煮熟   发酵   制成豆豉

功效分析

豆豉可以说是最早的化学合成药之一。在加工制作前，需先将大豆与麻黄、紫苏等拌合。麻黄、紫苏皆为辛温之品，具有较强的发汗作用，在与大豆相拌后，也就将它们的特性部分赋予了大豆，因而发酵而成的豆豉也具有了与麻黄、紫苏相类似的发汗功效，但作用相对温和。故对于故事中阎都督等上了年纪，不宜过度发汗的病人可以说是十分适宜。

Efficacy Analysis

Douchi is one of the earliest chemical synthetic drugs. Before processing, soya beans should be mixed with Mahuang (*Ephedra sinica*), Zisu (*Perilla frutescens*), etc. Mahuang and Zisu are pungent and warm products, which have strong diaphoretic effect. After being mixed with soya beans, they give some of their characteristics to soya beans, so fermented Douchi also has similar diaphoretic effect as Mahuang and Zisu, but relatively mild. Therefore, it is very suitable for patients like Governor Yan who are old and not suitable to sweat excessively.

通达病所媒药引
Drugs for Targeting

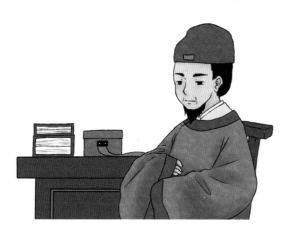

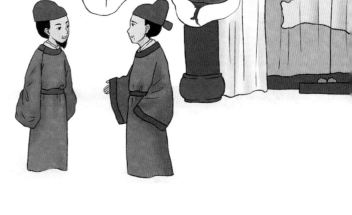

明朝洪武年间，浙江萧山有个叫楼英的郎中，出身医药世家，医术高明。

During the Hongwu Period of the Ming Dynasty, there lived a doctor named Lou Ying in Xiaoshan County, Zhejiang Province. He was born in a family of medicine and had excellent medical skills.

这年当朝皇后得了重病，明太祖心急如焚，遍请天下名医给皇后治病。楼英也应邀进宫。入宫后，打听皇后病情，见其所用皆是人参、鹿茸之品，料想马皇后必定已是病入膏肓难以救治。

When the empress of the Ming Dynasty fell ill, the worried emperor, Taizu called all the famous doctors to the imperial court. And Lou Ying was just one of them. At the palace, after Lou Ying had inquired about the empress's illness, he found that all the medicines used were ginseng and pilose antler, so he inferred that Empress Ma was surely beyond cure.

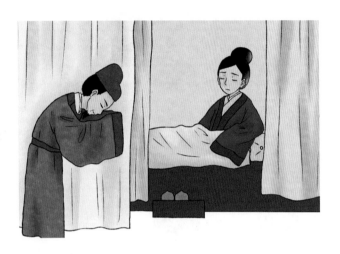

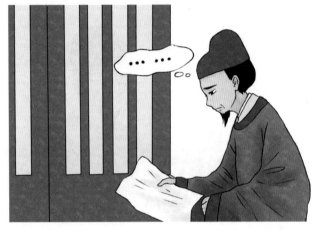

等到第二天，楼英跟着太监来到马皇后病榻前，仔细望闻问切一番后，皱着的眉头渐渐舒展开了。以楼英看来，马皇后只不过是多食引起脾胃不和，饮食积滞，只要用大黄、莱菔子这些极普通的药便可治愈。

The next day, Lou Ying followed the eunuch to Empress Ma's bedside. After careful examination through observing, questioning and pulse feeling, he unlocked his frown. Lou Ying diagnosed that Empress Ma's illness only resulted from the over intake of food and food stagnation due to the disharmony between the spleen and stomach. So the disease was curable with very common medicines such as rhubarb and radish seeds.

楼英疑惑太医院御医如云却怎会束手无策呢？于是他又将之前的药方拿出来斟酌起来。突然小有所悟：这些药无益无害，但恰合皇后凤体之贵，倘若用药低廉，一旦有闪失追究下来，定将大祸临头。

Lou Ying wondered why so many doctors of the Imperial Medical College were helpless. So he took out the previous prescription and studied carefully. Suddenly he realized that these drugs were neither useful nor harmful, but rare and expensive. It turned out that, considering the empress's honorable social position, no one would risk his life by using cheap medicines.

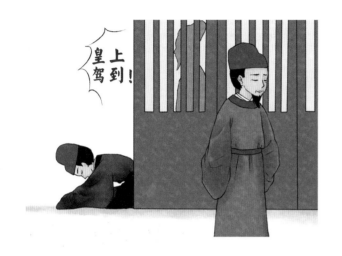

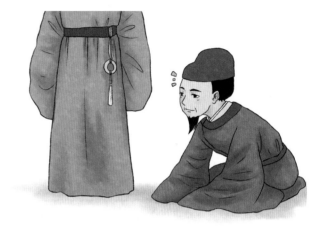

领悟了其中利害，楼英左思右想，也不敢贸然下笔了。就在他心中为难时，外面太监高声喊道："皇上驾到！"

叩拜之时，楼英见明太祖皇袍上有一块玉佩晶莹剔透，心中不禁一动：我何不用皇上玉佩做药引抬高身价？

Just as Lou Ying was hesitating, the eunuch outside shouted loudly, "Here comes His Majesty!"

While bowing down, Lou Ying caught a sight of a crystal-clear jade pendant on the Emperor Taizu's imperial robe, so he got an idea, "Why not use emperor's jade pendant as a medicinal usher to show the value of medicinal materials?"

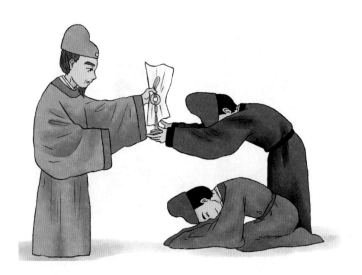

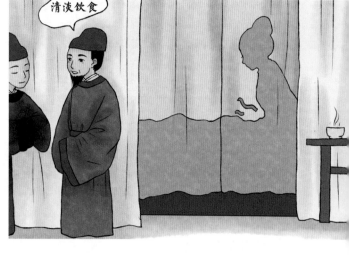

想到这儿，楼英心下安稳了，提笔写道：莱菔子三钱，皇上随身玉佩做药引。朱元璋看了，马上解下玉佩，连同药方一起递给太监。

Reassured, Lou Ying decisively wrote a prescription: "Three qian of radish seeds, with the emperor's jade pendant as a medicinal usher." The emperor read it, immediately took off the jade pendant, and handed to the eunuch the jade pendant along with the prescription.

不一会儿，太监将药抓来煎好，服侍马皇后服下。当晚，马皇后腹内"咕咕"作响，大便通畅，安稳地睡了一夜。第二天，楼英又让她进少许淡粥素菜。几日之后，马皇后便病体痊愈，行动如初了。

After a while, the eunuch took the medicine and served it to Empress Ma. In the evening, Empress Ma's abdomen "cooed" and her stods were smooth, and then she had a sound sleep all night. The next day, Lou Ying made her have some plain porridge with vegetables. A few days later, Empress Ma recovered and became as healthy as she used to be.

药引介绍
The Introduction of Medicinal Usher

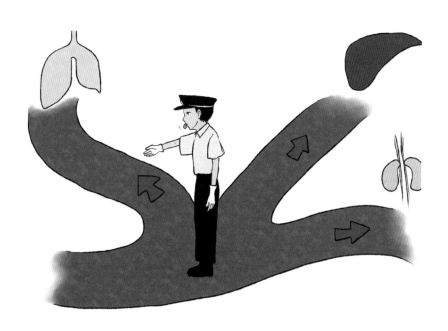

功效分析

故事中，玉佩作药引或许只是楼英巧妙抬高药价所作的一个"幌子"。不过，在中药理论中确有药引之说，这些药物能够引导其他药物到达病变部位或某一经脉，如中药中的牛膝，性趋下，能够引药下行治疗下焦疾病；白芷可引药达阳明经，治疗前额眉棱骨疼痛，以起到向导的作用，也被称为引经报使药。

Efficacy Analysis

In the story, the jade pendant, functioning as a medicinal usher, might only be Lou Ying's "quick wit" for raising the treatment cost. However, in the theory of traditional Chinese medicine, there is indeed the application of medicinal usher. These medications can accurately position other drugs to the lesion site or a certain meridian. For example, Niuxi (*Achyranthes bidentata*) can better treat lower energizer diseases by conducting medicines downward. Baizhi (*Angelica dahurica*) can lessen more effectively the pain in forehead eyebrow ridge bone by helping medicines to reach *yangming* channel (one of the meridians in traditional Chinese medicine), thus playing the role of "guide". That's why it is also known as channel conduction medicinals.

后记：
源于中药的
诺贝尔奖

Postscript:
The Nobel Prize from
Traditional Chinese
Medicine

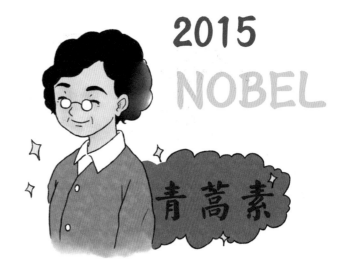

2015 年，中国科学家屠呦呦因从青蒿中提炼得到治疗疟疾的新型特效药——青蒿素，而获得了当年的诺贝尔生理学或医学奖。

In 2015, Chinese scientist Tu Youyou won the Nobel Prize in Physiology or Medicine for extracting artemisinin, a new specific drug for malaria treatment.

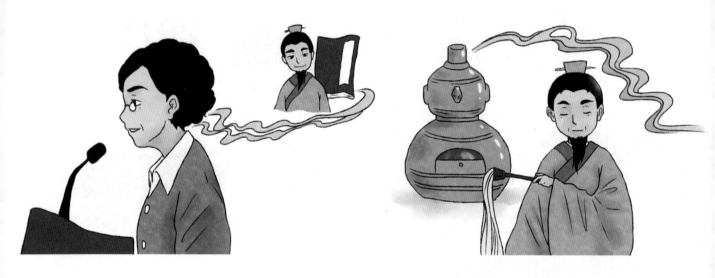

在发表获奖感言时，屠呦呦却坦言她提取青蒿素的灵感来源并非源于如今发达的现代技术，而是得益于一部古书——葛洪的《肘后备急方》。

In her award-winning speech, Tu Youyou frankly admitted that her inspiration for artemisinin extraction did not come from today's advanced modern technology, but from an ancient book, Ge Hong's *A Handbook of Prescriptions for Emergencies.*

葛洪是东晋时期著名的炼丹家、医学家，《肘后备急方》则是其代表性医学著作。

Ge Hong was a famous alchemist and medical expert in the Eastern Jin Dynasty, and *A Handbook of Prescriptions for Emergencies* was his representative works in medical field.

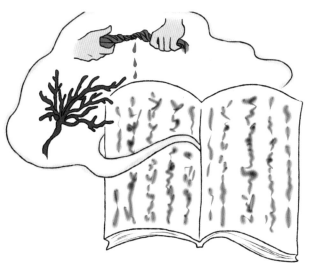

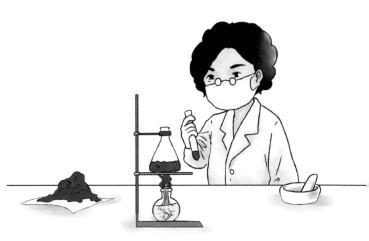

20世纪60年代，青蒿素的提取是世界公认的难题。而有一天，屠呦呦在翻看《肘后备急方》时，发现书中有这样一段记载："青蒿一握。以水二升渍，绞取汁。尽服之。"

In the 1960s, the extraction of artemisinin was regarded as a tough issue in the world. One day, when reading Ge Hong's book, Tu Youyou found a paragraph in the book that said, "Take fresh Qinghao (*Artemisia annua*), soak in clear water, wring it for juice, and take all the liquid."

屠呦呦便思考为何不用水煎，是害怕高温破坏青蒿的疗效吗？于是她和她的团队便将温度控制在60℃处理青蒿，最终获得青蒿素。

Tu Youyou wondered, "Why not boil it in the hot water? Is it because that the high temperature would lower the efficacy of Qinghao?" So she and her team tried keeping the temperature at 60℃ during the process and finally obtained artemisinin successfully.

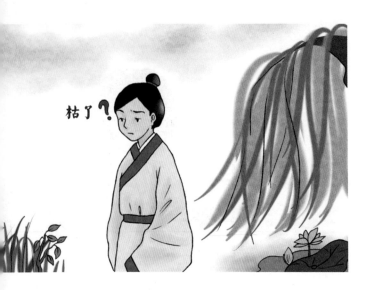

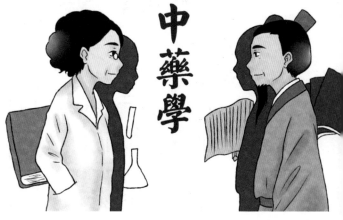

古人对于药物的解读并非通过现今完善的药理和动物实验，除了神农尝百草的试药精神外，更多的是来源于对植物生长特性的观察和考量。

Unlike modern doctors, the ancient people did not have perfect pharmacology and animal experiments for medical study. Apart from Shennong's spirit of testing herbs on his own body, they mainly gained knowledge through careful observation of plants' growth characteristics.

不可否认，古人对药物的认识有着其独到的智慧，融合中华传统文化的中医药理论后，构建了当今中药学的根基。这也是我们现代中医人所要不断探寻挖掘的，屠呦呦的获奖正是源自于此。

It is undeniable that the ancients had their own wisdom in understanding of drugs, and that the traditional Chinese medical theory, integrated with traditional Chinese culture, has laid the foundation of modern Chinese medicine. That is what we modern Chinese medicine practitioners must persistently explore; and that is what led Tu Youyou to the honorable prize.

55检